INSPIRATIONAL AROMATHERAPY

The Writings of Beverley Higham

BEVERLEY HIGHAM

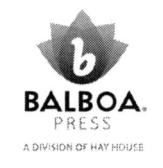

BALBOA
PRESS
A DIVISION OF HAY HOUSE

Copyright © 2015 Beverley Higham.

All rights reserved. No part of this book may be used or reproduced by any means, graphic, electronic, or mechanical, including photocopying, recording, taping or by any information storage retrieval system without the written permission of the publisher except in the case of brief quotations embodied in critical articles and reviews.

Balboa Press books may be ordered through booksellers or by contacting:

Balboa Press
A Division of Hay House
1663 Liberty Drive
Bloomington, IN 47403
www.balboapress.com
1 (877) 407-4847

Because of the dynamic nature of the Internet, any web addresses or links contained in this book may have changed since publication and may no longer be valid. The views expressed in this work are solely those of the author and do not necessarily reflect the views of the publisher, and the publisher hereby disclaims any responsibility for them.

The author of this book does not dispense medical advice or prescribe the use of any technique as a form of treatment for physical, emotional, or medical problems without the advice of a physician, either directly or indirectly. The intent of the author is only to offer information of a general nature to help you in your quest for emotional and spiritual well-being. In the event you use any of the information in this book for yourself, which is your constitutional right, the author and the publisher assume no responsibility for your actions.

Any people depicted in stock imagery provided by Thinkstock are models, and such images are being used for illustrative purposes only. Certain stock imagery © Thinkstock.

Print information available on the last page.

ISBN: 978-1-5043-2845-6 (sc)
ISBN: 978-1-5043-2846-3 (e)

Balboa Press rev. date: 03/05/2015

Inspirational Aromatherapy –
The writings of Beverley Higham

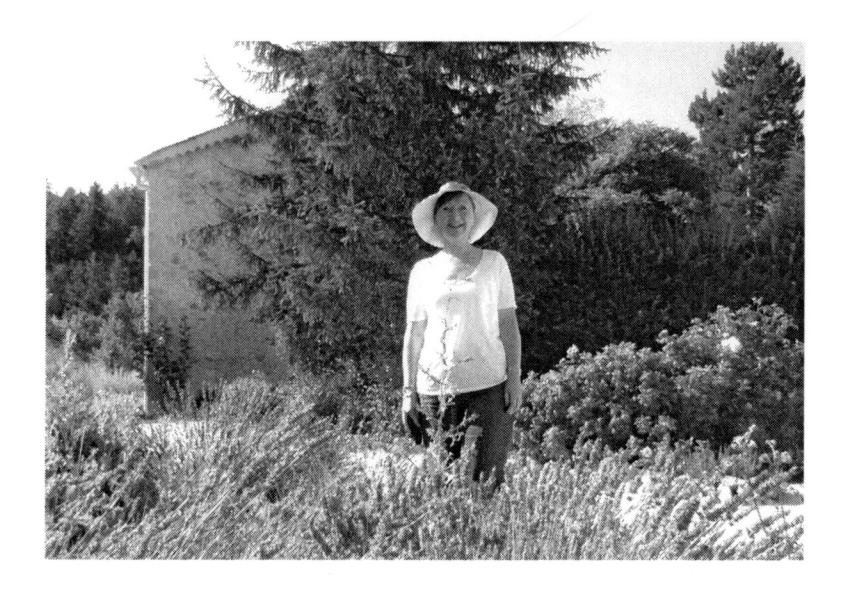

Beverley Higham is a highly acclaimed Aromatherapist and international teacher with a vast experience of Aromatherapy and product development. She has a BA in Education and is a member of IFPA. She is co-founder and creative director of Potionshop UK a range of natural organic face, body and spa products. She is also a Lecturer and course Manager at Wigan and Leigh College.

I would like to thank Jane Hatton for introducing me to Aromatherapy many years ago; it has truly blessed my life. I would also like to thank all of my wonderful students (you know who you are) for making my career such an amazing one. My Colleagues and mentors along the way, far too many to mention but my personal development and educational journey would never have happened without them. Debra and Jim Atherton for allowing me to join them for my first visit to Provence. Jonathan Hinde and Malte Hozzel from Oshadhi essential oils. Bob Harris, Rhiannon Harris Lewis for the aromatic adventures. Angela Mahandru and Choice Health magazine for encouraging my writing. My business partner Bernie Mulligan for her absolute belief in me.

Most of all I would like to thank my wonderful parents Brian and Joan Wilson for their love and endless support and my partner Mohammed Dad.

Dedicated to Scarlett and Tommy-Lee, everything I do is for you.

Inspirational Aromatherapy

My interest in plants came from my Mother and her Parents. My earliest childhood memories are of the smell and colour of the wall flowers that lined my grandfather's driveway. He also had a green house full of geraniums and fusias. I loved to sit in the green house and watch him tend to the flowers. When I was five years old we moved away from my Grandparents home and went to live close to the Manchester ship canal. This was a highly built up area surrounded by council owned properties and concrete flats. Far from gardens of flowers or the countryside. My Mother had a wealth of knowledge about plants and wild life and my interest continued with the urban safaris she took me and my friends on through the suburbs of Manchester finding nature amongst the flag stones and deserted stretches of land. She turned our walks into botany lessons and magical adventures where we would return with pussy willow, apple blossom and frogs spawn. I grew passionate about wild flowers, which I studied intently and knew all their Latin names. It was a strange pastime for a young Girl.

I guess that my inspiration came from those early days, but it wasn't until I reached my twenties that I discovered Aromatherapy!

I was a beauty therapist and training to teach my subject. A colleague who had worked on cruise ships was giving a small micro teach to the group about Aromatherapy. I listened to her intently in fact I was so spellbound that I felt a light go on in my head and I suddenly realised that this was what I was born to do!

I found a course in London and away I went. I have never looked back, my life is filled with aroma and I have met such wonderful people and been to the most amazing places through my work with essential oils. I have won awards and accolades for my work but most of all it has brought me to this point, where I can share my stories with you. Many of you reading this book will have been on aromatic adventures with me; those of you who have not yet studied with me will (I hope) enjoy this book and my teachings. Knowledge is a gift and all that is not given is lost, so please enjoy my stories and recipes.

This is not an academic text book or a referenced study. It is the result of my experiences in the world of aromatherapy and an account of some of my case studies. The recipes in here are my suggestions and much of the information is anecdotal. If you are on medication or in poor health please check with your doctor before use or seek out a professional Aromatherapist. None of my suggestions are to replace modern medicine. It is very important that you always seek the advice of a physician if you have any health problems. Nature is very powerful and if you are on medication you need to be sure that any essential oils you may use will not interact adversely with your medication. Essential oils must always be diluted and never taken internally.

Enjoy your aromatic adventures.

Beverley Higham.

Contents

Chapter 1.	Aromatherapy is more than a smelly treatment	1
Chapter 2.	Aromatherapy for healers	7
Chapter 3.	The Aromatic Woman what do I need to Grow	14
Chapter 4.	Aromatherapy in Pregnancy	19
Chapter 5.	Aromatherapy for babies and young children	25
Chapter 6.	Aromatherapy for the Menopause	31
Chapter 7.	Aromatherapy in the Home	35
Chapter 8.	Aromatherapy and oral hygiene	39
Chapter 9.	Cleopatra's beauty secrets	42
Chapter 10.	The oils of love	48
Chapter 11.	Sense-ology - Treatments that touch deeper	51
Chapter 12.	Destination Provence	55

Chapter 1

Aromatherapy is more than a smelly treatment

Aromatherapy is more than a smelly treatment - it is the controlled use of essential oils extracted from aromatic plants by a process known as distillation.

Many people think of Aromatherapy as just another form of massage or a Beauty treatment with nothing more than superficial benefits but it is so much more than that!

The word Aroma means smell and therapy means treatment - so our nose plays a vital role in the process and this is where the greatest impact can be made. As we inhale pleasing fragrant aromas the cilia in our olfactory bulb at the back of the nose picks up the tiny molecules and like keys turning in locks the pathway to the neuro transmitters in the brain are opened and "pow!" we have the real effect of aromatherapy just as it was intended. Suddenly our body feels the soothing effects as our endorphins and encephalin are released, our limbic system transports us to lavender fields from long forgotten memories or puts us in the Rose scented arms of our Grandmothers as children once more. Essential oils can stimulate the limbic system which is the oldest part of our brain and the seat of all emotion. This is where the real treatment starts. Aromatherapy is a body, mind and spirit treatment that is what makes it truly holistic. By spirit we mean the charisma, personality and the essential part of what makes a person who they are and how they interact with life. We often refer to the term "high spirited", or "low in spirit". Aromatherapy can revive the spirit. As just like the petals of the flowers we obtain essential oils from, we humans open and close Depending on our moods and emotions. We have such synergy with essential oils because we are part of the same whole, life itself.

Aromatherapy is a powerful tool for developing peace of mind when our outer world is in turmoil, composure when we are steering through troubled times and vitality when our get up and go has got up and gone! Aromatherapy can support us through the changing times of our lives from childhood with growing pains, anxiety and night terrors that accompany this stage in our lives. Soothing, mothering Roman Chamomile, familiar and comforting lavender and fruity uplifting mandarin help children who are often never considered to be suffering from "stress"! It is not just adults that experience this dreaded condition and the effects of relationship break ups and the saga that can develop from disruption in our lives. This is when Aromatherapy can support those moments in time. Children should be encouraged to choose their own essential oils by smelling the lid of the bottle and allowing their tiny nose to draw its own conclusion as to what is best for them. Children enjoy fruity and flowery smells. I recently prepared a roller ball essential oil blend for a friend for her ten year old son. How should he use it she asked me? Knowing how intelligent her son was I told her to ask him how he wanted to use it? She returned the following week stating with a smile that he had applied the tiny roll on, around his nipples and belly button!

Oh how intuitive I replied, his heart and sacral chakra's, what a wise child. (He too was feeling the break-up of his separated parents and inner wisdom was being his guide as to where to put the blend.) It could just have been him having fun, but that is the beauty of Aromatherapy it's gentle, safe and effective in the right hands and so much more than a smelly treatment".

The turbulent teens and hormonal disruption!

We are all affected by the ups and downs and rhythms of life, from physical and physiological changes as we develop and grow through to the slower process as we reach peak and hit the gentle downward slope into the twilight and evening of our lives which brings with it new experiences.

As we reach our teenage years our bodies respond to the flood of hormones in many ways. Mood and emotion disrupts the quiet child we once knew and in some cases the terrible teen emerges.

PMT or PMS is a common collection of symptoms from food cravings, tearfulness, cramps and breast tenderness. Sometimes these cramps are so debilitating that they can stop a young woman in her tracks and keep her from work and study. Using essential oils throughout the cycle can prevent or at least soften these symptoms. 12 days before the period is due is a good time to start using a prepared blend. Aromatherapy really is more than a smelly treatment which helps soothes changeable moods and swinging emotions Bergamot and Geranium balancing and uplifting, dissolving depressive thoughts and generating positivity. Rose and Clary sage help to tone and regulate the cycle, reducing stress and easing cramps. The oils can be most beneficial for calming monthly anxiety when inhaled from a tissue or smelling strip. For more physical symptoms applied in a base oil or lotion to the abdomen and lower back at the onset of discomfort or if periods are regular, use as a preventative a day before the period is due.

Teenagers can be prone to breakouts of pimples and pustules. Just at the time when they are developing their image and are at a very self-conscious stage in their development and trying to find their identity and personal image.

Therefore when blending essential oils to treat the skin we need to remember the emotional effect problem skin can have and use uplifting aromas which sooth the mood and the blemish!

Lavender, bergamot and Geranium are ideal in a calendula and Grapeseed base for mild acne and general hormonal break outs. Tea tree and lavender in a cleansing gel assist good skin hygiene and equally in aloe Vera gel make a good spot treatment.

Many teenagers have eczema, dry rough patches of skin that are irritating and unsightly (in their eyes). The skin is said to be a flag ship for underlying emotions so needs tender care just like our tender teen. Using an organic base cream add avocado oil rich and nourishing, it takes the redness out of the skin, calendula and chamomile are also anti-inflammatory they soften and reduce inflammation even further, frankincense and lavender rejuvenate and restore the condition of the skin by healing and repairing the skins natural balance.

Negativity and dark moods can also strike during the turbulent teens, relationships are difficult and angry outbursts are all too often. To help to create harmony in the home use a natural room spray, rose water with rose geranium leaves a cleansing refreshing aroma and attracts loving harmony to the environment. Juniperberry on the doormat creates a natural aromatic barrier to protect the home leaving negativity and other troubles we can bring into the home - outside! Like an aromatic sheep dip, as we walk over the aromatic doormat we cleanse ourselves of the emotional clutter that we have picked up throughout the day. Its hard being a teenager as we all know, we were once in our teens but having aromatherapy at hand can help the whole family cope with the turbulent teens.

Create a simple room fragrance spray;

100ml of floral water such as rose water.
10 drops of lavender essential oil
10 drops of juniperberry.

Shake well before use and then use as a room spray to cleanse the air and environment.

Chapter 2

Aromatherapy for healers

If you are a healer then you are passionate about helping people. So are essential oils. Essential oils are safe natural chemical messengers that can deliver messages deep into the body and stimulate the body providing support for the body to heal itself. Essential oils when respected are not harmful. It is the people using them that are the danger! Aromatherapy is the controlled use of essential oils, I emphasise the word controlled! It's how we use them that are important and how we educate our clients to use them. In the UK we do not recommend the internal use of essential oils. This method is employed by Doctors only, in some European countries such as France.

The subtle use of essential oils can restore balance and harmony to the body and mind and produce a restorative effect that is quite astounding. One of my most popular blends, Prime Time Plus is a subtle blend of essential oils in Aloe Vera, jojoba and rosehip; it's a blend of 4 essential oils, flowers, fruit and herb essences. When applied externally (dermal application) it results in the total eradication of debilitating symptoms associated with the female cycle (for most women). It also has an amazing effect on the skin, I have witnessed a severe case of psoriasis subside in less than a week following the application of the gel based solution. After 25 years working with essential oils I am still astounded by their magic and mystery for absorption we are told is so minimal from dermal application and yet the results can be phenomenal.

My healing oil emergency kit. 1

Lavender – Calming
Chamomile - soothing
Tea tree - fortifying
Eucalyptus - expanding
Bergamot - uplifting
Geranium - balancing
Clary sage - relaxing
Rose - loving
Lemon grass/Lime - revitalising
Juniper berry - cleansing

My healing oil emotional kit 2.

Spikenard - releasing
Helichrysum - healing
Cedarwood Himalayan - strengthening
Sandalwood - releasing
Neroli - comforting
Frankincense - easing

Lavender - a universal healer, intuitive oil that massages the nervous system from the inside. Soothing everything it comes into contact with. The most powerful of all healing oils. A strong violet healing energy. In healing it can be used to fragrance the room or diluted on the hands before treatment or given to the client on a tissue for inhalation. It has the ability to heal external wounds and stimulate inner healing due to its chemical make-up.

Chamomile - I longed for this soothing healer after I had had surgery. My body cried out for this pain relieving oil. When combined with Lavender they increase each other's healing ability. Chamomile is full of anti-inflammatory chemicals that quench any form of overheating. It's gentle and safe. Calming and deeply soothing. It allows us to nurture our client's inner child.

Tea tree - is more than an antiseptic. It is a pillar of strength to the weak. It's a rock and a shield of protection. It gives strength to fight any battles on a physical and emotional level. It has a deep ancient wisdom used by the wisest people on the planet the Aborigines of Australia the Bungalung tribe.

Eucalyptus - A wonderful penetrating, cooling oil. Its chemical composition allows it to reach deep into the body opening up the airways and cooling inflammation. A profoundly healing oil and "opener" of the body.

Bergamot - Refreshing and versatile. This beautiful oil has an amazing ability to balance on so many levels. From skin, to bladder, to emotions and the hormonal system, this is a remarkable gift from nature and one of my favourite oils. Uplifting the spirit and restoring hope and possibility.

Geranium - balancing and harmonising. Gentle oil that improves the general circulation. The natural flow of the body. Toning and supportive especially to the female system. The oil also encourages inner creativity and beauty.

Clary -sage - A very powerful oil with stress relieving qualities. Uplifting yet at the same time relaxing to a weary body and aiding sleep when you have trouble drifting off. Clary-sage is also great for the respiratory system relieving tightness in the chest and aiding the breath. Clary sage is also an oil that accompanies the female on her journey through her cycle of life from puberty and menstrual tension, through child birth to menopause.

Rose - Subtle soothing rose, bringing peace of mind and ease for the heart and mind. Broken spirits and grief are enveloped in the soft aroma and nurtured back to health. I like to use Lavender, rose geranium and Rose makes a beautiful synergy. Especially when coping with change.

Juniper berry - This oil cleanses the mind of emotional clutter. It wards off negativity and is highly protective oil. Cleansing and refreshing, clearing and detoxifying physically and emotionally. One of my all-time favourites.

Occasionally we need oils to work on a much higher level. When we are stuck in a certain place on an emotional level or held back by the baggage from the past that we cannot leave behind then we need that extra strength that comes with the following oils.

Spikenard - this is biblical oil and the one used by Mary Magdalene to massage the feet of Jesus before his crucifixion. It is a resolver of pain and relieves deep emotional blockages. It is said to regulate the heart beat and being a relative of valerian it relaxes the mind and helps us to sleep better. Native to the Himalayan region this plant is known as the flowering rhizome for it is the root that gives us this remarkable healing oil. Its earthy fragrance is instantly grounding and relaxing although its aroma is not appealing to everyone. As I always tell my students "follow your nose and let your intuition guide you".

Helichrysum - for inner and outer bruising. This essential oil known as Immortelle is healing both physically and emotionally. When combined with Lavender it is miraculous for external bruising. Used emotionally it is healing to our mind and brings peace and balance. A protective and restorative oil which blends well with other oils such as rose. Its spice like aroma is intensely soothing and musk like. This is definitely an oil for any aromatic first aid kit.

Himalayan Cedarwood - this is one of my all-time favourite oils. Its rich aroma has an ancient strength. It expands the breath and supports the circulatory system. The great temples of Lebanon were said to be built with Himalayan cedar. This oil is helpful when wishing to strengthen the connection with the divine. I first came upon it at a conference many years ago, a world Aromatherapy conference which took place at Warwick University. It was an inspirational event. At the trade show I was handed a small wooden box containing a tiny collection of oils. They were the oils of the Himalayas and I was totally mesmerised by their fragrance. The box was a gift from one of the traders and I still have it today. Phoenix oils thank you.

Sandalwood - this oil is favoured by many it has a sweet gentle aroma and brings instant calm. It is a great stress reliever and stills the mind. An aid to meditation, antispasmodic to the muscles and soothing to the skin. It is a first choice when stress is present and I like to blend it with Basil and Lavender. It is highly antiseptic and has an affinity with the throat chakra. Blended in carrier oil it can be applied to the throat (externally) to aid communication.

Neroli- Orange blossom from the bitter orange tree. An exotic aroma with earthy undertones a natural anti-depressant and uplifter of the spirits. This oil is excellent for anxiety and post natal depression. It blends beautifully with Frankincense or for a truly abundant synergy try Neroli, bitter orange and Petitgrain. 3 oils from the same tree. The oils of abundance, one tree that gives us 3 beautiful gifts. The blossom Neroli, twigs and leaves Petitgrain and the fruit bitter orange.

Frankincense - I love Indian Frankincense Boswellia serrata. Frankincense is a timeless fragrance. Recognised by many as a holy fragrance. It induces a relaxed state of mind and aids deep breathing. The oil is said to aid transitions in life and release us from the chains of the past. It is helpful for grief and loss. This beautiful essential oil aids healing on many levels.

Aromatherapy the use of essential oils is a truly remarkable therapy that can be combined with so many other forms of healing and most of all Aromatherapists can empower their clients with home care products for self-administration. All it takes is education of how to use the oils safely. I believe Aromatherapy is for everyone.

Chapter 3

The Aromatic Woman what do I need to Grow

I am privileged to be a woman, yet the true privilege of a life time we are told is to be who you are!

As a woman we have the opportunity to assist the universe in the miracle of creating new life and those who have not had children still have the qualities and abilities to nurture and be guardians of the race.

As an Aromatherapist I realise the close link between plant healing and human wellbeing. We humans are so similar to plants in many ways. As women we need regular attention, nurturing, admiration, we open and close depending upon the mood and emotion, the weather or time of day and the general environment. This along with our chemical make-up links us to the plant kingdom. As we too are fragrant aromatic beings.

Our life would not have been possible without life giving plants - life giving life from the beginning of time, evolving together as Mother Nature worked her miracle. We can encourage and continue our personal growth with Aromatherapy; beautiful essential oils help us to grow. They help us to expand physically and emotionally, the power of aroma can be experienced on so many levels.

Flower oils touch the soul - a symbol of feminine in nature, sensual, chemical messengers carrying the secret of life.

As women we need to recognise how beautiful and vibrant we are and match our chosen aroma/ perfume to our mood to increase this vibrancy.

Case study -

There is a feminine force that I have witnessed many times as a practitioner and teacher of aromatherapy. I once taught a young girl who had been expelled from her studies by many of the other tutors at her College. She was seen as aggressive and volatile. Every one told her she was useless and would never make it as a Therapist. I asked her to join my class and I watched her blossom in the presence of natural products and caring colleagues. One day I asked her to bring in a client to work on as a case study. She brought in an old work colleague of mine who had recently undergone surgery to have both breasts removed as a result of cancer. Previously she had had a hysterectomy and had undergone chemotherapy. The client lay on the treatment couch smiling although all of what physically makes us a woman had been removed and her hair and lashes fallen out. With Doctors permission to treat her, I witnessed this lady be brought back to full bloom. Like a dormant bulb yet full of possibilities this lady blossomed again over a series of aromatherapy treatments, in the hands of a nurturing therapist. Cancer is a part of many people's lives and we are all fearful of it but with modern medicine and complementary therapy we can bloom again. In this case study two people were healed, the client and the Therapist. As we age we seek out anti-ageing treatments. Yet why are we so afraid go growing older?

Margaret Maury said about ageing "only the unknown enemy is to be feared" She also stated "to live, to be alive, means to be in motion, to evolve to transform one's self". Like a good wine we mature into wisdom, knowledge and grace if we allow ourselves to embrace change and learn from it. Essential oils are the result of the distillation process, the plant giving itself up to be turned into the liquid gold we capture in our tiny bottles, each drop part of an alchemical healing process "Aromatherapy". If we imagine life to be the process of distillation then we to can find our essential self in our maturing years.

As we travel through the many changing phases of our life as females Aromatherapy can support us. My personal choice for this journey is listed below;

1. Mandarin - this is known as the children's oil in France. Its fruity aroma dissolves tiny tantrums and the refreshing aroma cools hysterical outbursts.

INSPIRATIONAL AROMATHERAPY

Great for tiny toddlers. Always use highly diluted in vegetable based oil such as sunflower oil. 1 drop in 10 ml for massage or 1 drop on a tissue for inhalation.

2. Bergamot and Geranium - the onset of menstruation can cause many symptoms from painful periods, bloating and mood swings. These two balancing and uplifting essential oils harmonise perfectly to alleviate monthly symptoms. 2 drops of each in 15 ml of sunflower oil can be massaged into the abdomen and lower back for comfort or 1 drop of each inhaled from a tissue. For stressful and emotional symptoms try diluting 3 drops of each in a cup full of milk and swishing in the bath for a nice soak. These oils will carry us through our prime time years.

3. Neroli- deeply relaxing and gentle oil that help us to unwind and recharge. It's gentle enough to use after pregnancy to prevent or ease postnatal depression. Diluted in rose-hip and jojoba oil it can help to diminish stretch marks. An ideal all round female oil.

4. Jasmine and Vetiver- when our twilight years arrive our body needs the extra grounding and confidence building aromas of these exotic plants. The aphrodisiac Jasmine rekindles fading thoughts of femininity and vetiver cools our body and holds us together. They can be blended with lime essential

oil for a refreshing cleansing effect keeping our energy field free from negativity. Apply diluted in nourishing base oil such as sweet almond oil. Work on the upper body especially close to the solar plexus.

5. Frankincense - as we approach the final years of our journey and that journey may be long. We can vaporise Frankincense for its soothing, calming and meditative attributes. It moves us forward like the kings and queens of Egypt, to an afterlife of riches. It quenches anxiety that often fills us with fear of ageing and ultimately the end of our physical life.

We live on a very aromatic planet and we have an abundance of natural plant oils that are available today. Take time to find an Aromatherapist or invest in a good book on the subject and let your nose lead you to wellbeing.

Chapter 4

Aromatherapy in Pregnancy

There are many benefits that can be found with Aromatherapy during pregnancy. It is important to be cautious if you have not previously used essential oils before you became pregnant. The general advice is to avoid the use of essential oils in the first trimester and avoid certain strong oils due to their chemical make-up. Essential oils which are rich in phenols and useful for fighting infection will be too strong for the sensitive and delicate skin of the pregnant woman. These stimulating oils should be avoided throughout the whole of the pregnancy. It is also important to avoid essential oils which may be photosensitive as during pregnancy women have raised melanin stimulating hormone levels.

If you have used essential oils before and have no history of miscarriage then with professional guidance both massage and aromatherapy can be very beneficial throughout your pregnancy and especially during the early stages of labour. When using essential oils it is important to remember that there are now two people who will benefit. Mother and growing child. If Mother is relaxed and healthy then so will the baby be relaxed and healthy. I always recommend a lower dosage of essential oils in a blend during pregnancy but we must remember that the Mothers body can still metabolise as normal and has an extra layer of fat surrounding the baby who again is safely supported in its own protective bubble.

Fruit and flower oils are favoured for their gentle stress relieving properties and uplifting qualities. Always use high grade essential oils from a reputable supplier and preferably organic or wild crafted, only the best will do at this time. Therapeutic essential oils of a high quality can present very little hazard in comparison to low grade or synthetic oils.

The small amount of essential oil that actually accesses the Mothers skin is a minuscule amount and there have been no recorded instances where harm has been caused using aromatherapy massage during pregnancy.

Often pregnancy carries a stigma of a no go zone for Therapists. But this is the time when Holistic Therapies can provide tremendous support up to and during labour and beyond.

The main thing to remember is that being pregnant is not an illness. I taught Aromatherapy all through my pregnancy and my daughter continued to receive Aromatherapy from conception until the day of her baby's birth.

The following oils are the ones I find beneficial. Always seek professional advice before having an Aromatherapy treatment and ensure you use the services of a highly trained Therapist.

Lavender (high altitude) is stress relieving and relaxing both physically and emotionally and this oil is said to be safe during pregnancy. Much research has been done to verify that high altitude Lavendula angusitifolia is a safe oil in pregnancy. It is useful for anxiety, tension, aches and pains or insomnia.

Chamomile (chamaemelum Nobile) roman chamomile is a gentle flowering herbaceous plant with comforting, soothing qualities. It eases discomfort and relaxes the body and mind. It is a mild pain reliever and therefore can ease aches and pains.

Mandarin (citrus reticulata) is uplifting and refreshing. A mood lifting fragrance. This can be used when energy is low. It is also a good oil to use along with lavender in a carrier oil to keep the skin soft and supple and prevent stretch marks.

Bergamot (citrus bergamia) is also a good oil for its stress relieving properties during pregnancy. Avoid using it on exposed skin when out in the sun as it is photosensitive, yet this oil is very emotionally supportive and helpful for minor urinary tract disorders which can occur during pregnancy. Vaporising the oil in the atmosphere is a safe and pleasant way of using Bergamot.

Spearmint (mentha spicata) is a pleasant essential oil to sniff if nausea is a problem. It is gentler than peppermint but equally refreshing and carminative.

Frankincense (Boswellia carteri) is oil that calms and regulates the breathing. It is good for reducing anxiety especially when used with Ylang Ylang (cananga odorata). Frankincense is also supportive to the skin and can be used with the lavender and mandarin in a body oil. Ylang Ylang as mentioned is good for stress and anxiety and nervous tension, it is however hypotensive reducing blood pressure so bare this in mind if you already have low blood pressure.

Always use very low doses of essential oils as a little is often better than a lot.

2 drops of essential oil to 10 ml of vegetable oil for massage and 5 drops if using in an average sized bath, diluted in milk first. Milk emulsifies the oil so that it does not irritate sensitive body areas as you soak in the bath. To inhale from a tissue drip 2 drops on to a tissue or handkerchief. This will be adequate to inhale and never take essential oils internally.

A gentle Aromatherapy massage or aromatic bath will be soothing and beneficial throughout pregnancy. As you get closer to the due date for the birth your therapist can create blends for you to take into the labour ward with you. Most hospitals now also have essential oils for expectant Mothers to use during the early stages of labour. A warm bath with lavender and rose will relax the body and ease pain and anxiety. Once labour is established a blend of lavender and chamomile will ease pain. Once the cervix is fully dilated Clary- sage can be added to the lavender and chamomile blend to aid and support contractions. Clary- sage (salvia sclarea) should only be used in the very late stage of labour under the advice of your midwife and Aromatherapist.

Having a familiar aroma present at the baby's birth will be reassuring for the new-born for experts say that their sense of smell begins in the womb. Keeping everyone calm at this special time is key and aromatherapy has the potential to do this.

Under the advice of her Aromatherapist, Mum can continue to use essential oils at home by vaporising them to soothe emotions or adding a few drops of a recommended essential oil to her bath to eases stress and encourage healing. Good old Lavender is always top of the list but a variety of essential oils can be used. It's important to stick to the gentle safe oils at this time especially if breast feeding.

Lavender - stress relieving, calming and relaxing
Chamomile - soothing and pain relieving
Geranium- balancing the mood and emotions.
Rose - healing and toning
Neroli- anti-depressant
Orange- uplifting and energising
Bergamot- refreshing and normalising
Ylang Ylang - reduces anxiety

Aromatherapy is a general restorative treatment. Always choose an Aromatherapist with specialised training in Pregnancy and antenatal care there are many wonderful Therapists out there.

Chapter 5

Aromatherapy for babies and young children

We all benefit from pleasant aromas and Babies and young children are no different their early memories will be rich with aroma. Aromatherapy is linked with the olfactory system, which is described as the seat of all emotion; therefore aroma massage when performed safely can benefit both parent and child. It can be as simple as vaporising subtle fragrances in the home or adding a single drop of a gentle floral essential oil diluted in a little vegetable oil in the bath.

New babies have a whole world of new experiences awaiting them. Their skins are sensitive when they arrive in a world where the watery protection they had in their mother's womb has been replaced by an array of new chemicals and sensations. Their skin can become red and irritated - this is normal, as the new-born skin is like an antenna in the new world. Organic olive oil is best for dry baby skin and has been recommended by midwives for many years although recent research suggests that it may dry the skin further. Therefore cold pressed Sunflower or Grapeseed oil is suitable and avocado oil if the skin is excessively irritated. Use sparsely and on a small area to start with. Vegetable based oils are rich and nourishing to the skin. As baby gets older about 6 weeks add a little Calendula oil to the Base oil. This will improve the nourishing effects of the chosen base oil and sooth any minor irritation from dry patches or what is known as milk rash which can appear on the face, scalp, neck and chest. It's more common in boy babies and known as baby acne. This soon disappears so don't worry, it can look unsightly especially just before or after a feed. The skin will improve in no time at all. Once your baby is 6 weeks old a drop of chamomile or lavender can be introduced to the massage blend. Lavender is a gentle essential oil which is calming and soothing. Chamomile is relaxing, comforting and pain relieving. When these two oils are combined they increase the healing capacity of each other. Minor symptoms such as colic, teething and over tiredness can be eased with aromatherapy in a safe and effective way, but use in very small quantities with babies and young children. For babies under 1 year use 1 drop maximum and highly diluted in base oil. Avoid using essential oils in the first 6 weeks of a child's life.

Other ailments that may present themselves are coughs and colds, sniffles and general chesty mucous conditions. Vaporising frankincense in the environment is a safe effective treatment for all the family. It's anti-septic and anti-viral properties make it ideal, plus its calming and soothing to both body and mind. The stronger oils such as eucalyptus should not be used on the very young as they are far too powerful.

My favourite macerated oil is calendula. You may have gathered this as I mention it a lot. It's ideal for severe nappy rash it works like a miracle for taking away reddened inflamed skin. My grandson had a terrible rash and spots when he was 7 months. Little blisters on his knees and hands which were made worse by the fact that he was crawling. The Doctor thought it was chicken pox? I massaged calendula into the painful blisters and within a couple of days they had reduced considerably and the inflammation had gone down.

My ideal children's blend is a highly dilute blend of chamomile, lavender, geranium and mandarin just one drop of each in 50 ml of base oil such as sunflower. Use only a little of this each time (5 ml) and store it in a dark labelled bottle in a cool dark place. This blend is suitable for many childhood ailments. Children suffer from aches and pains, stresses and strains and a soothing massage always helps. Try massaging the feet and legs or the back. Children love massage. Gentle clockwise abdominal massage may help tummy ache with mandarin or sweet orange and chamomile? If your child is feeling stressed due to starting school or nursery try lavender or tea tree just one drop on a tissue this will soothe the nervous system and provide a welcome aromatic reminder that you are not far away. Linking aromas to memory is what we all do.

Case study;

Mother and baby Spa.

Tommy first visited the spa when he was 6 weeks old. To Tommy the Spa is a place of tranquillity and deep relaxation. The sound of the waves crashing on a tropical beach and the beautiful faces smiling at him are mesmerising, not to mention the fascinating low lighting and floral displays that tantalise one so young with curiosity. In fact Tommy has really been visiting the spa since his conception so the familiar environment will be a pleasant memory from the womb psychologists will tell us and I would agree.

Tommy never cries even when it is almost time for his bottle. The Spa environment is one he enjoys and is replenished by. Tranquillity is what a young child needs in this busy world of entertainment, TV, movies and video games or x boxes I believe they are called. A young child is exposed to so much stimulation in the modern world and to escape to the Spa is a sanctuary to both Mother and Child.

Mum has a coconut lomi lomi massage or this week a stress relieving body exfoliation and body wrap. The subtle aromas further stimulate Tommy's interest, being an aromatic baby in the sense that his birth involved the use of rose and lavender oil and Grandma massages him with organic olive oil and calendula which he highly recommends.

The environment is a tonic with all its embracing, comforting ingredients that a young child needs. Play and stimulating activities will always be in his life but to grow up with the ability to relax, meditate and enjoy calm surrounding without being "bored" is what we should aim to develop in our children. I believe that we entertain our young minds to the point of exhaustion so that children and teenagers expect us to continue to entertain them because to them alone time is boredom.

Tommy's mum has a 45 minute treatment, Tommy remains nearby and is cared for in the arms of his familiar therapist, who notices his forehead is a little dry. Luckily he has his organic olive oil with him. Whilst mum is treated to a massage Tommy has his own oil massaged onto his tiny forehead and surrenders to the peaceful surroundings. He has tried to stay awake and keep an eye on mum but its far to nice here at the spa his second home.

One day he may open a spa of his own he thinks. Tommy is looking forward to being a little older as he is then going to have an aromatherapy massage, but for now it is enough to enjoy the fragrance and benefit from the skin nourishing olive and calendula oil.

Baby's skin is very sensitive to the new environment after birth and due to the fact that they don't produce sebum to protect and nourish the skin, it is important to ensure that the newborn skin does not dry out. Always patch test any new massage oil (natural organic vegetable oil) on a small area of your babies skin before use and use only the best quality.

Mother and baby Spas are becoming popular. We need to remember that our children are just like we are and they pick up on our feelings when we are under stress. They need love and hugs but most of all but they need time and space to be quiet so that they can grow into wonderful whole human beings.

Toddler tantrums.

It's not easy being a toddler. There is so much of the world to explore and lack of communication can be a problem. Toddlers are prone to tiny tantrums. The perfect blend for a toddler would always include Mandarin as it is extremely calming for children. It reduces hysteria and anxiety. I developed a beautiful blend for babies and young children during my time in Clinical practice. Children love sweet flowery fruity fragrances. Mandarin, chamomile, geranium, lavender and a drop of sweet marjoram. This blend in sunflower and calendula macerated oil is ideal for a host of physical and emotions symptoms that children frequently experience. As I suggest earlier. It has as a side action the ability to ease teething pain and relax little ones, helping to cool and calm. If you have not got any essential oils at hand the best way to calm a toddler tantrum is to break the skin of a large orange and roll it towards them. The oil is released from the essential oil cavities in the peel and as the aroma meets the tiny nose you will notice instant calm.

Chapter 6

Aromatherapy for the Menopause

The menopause marks the end of the physical reproductive phase of a woman's life: in most cases it begins around the age of 45 and ends by 55 years of age although this can vary.

During this time women may experience changes such as:

- Body fat from the hips and thighs redistributed to the stomach and back.
- Hair, nails and skin become dry without the softening effects of oestrogen.
- Night sweats and hot flushes.
- feeling more emotional! Weepy and having a poor self- image.

Aromatherapy can be beneficial for these distressing and unpleasant symptoms - below is a list of the oils I have found most useful:

Vetiver (vetiveria zizanioides)

In my experience this oil, known in India as the 'oil of tranquillity ', can be highly beneficial when night sweats are disrupting normal sleep patterns. Cooling and grounding, it can act as a sedative to the nervous system. It blends well with clary-sage and sandalwood and aids restful sleep.

Petitgrain (citrus aurantium var amara)

This is useful for emotional transitions caused by the menopause. Blended with Frankincense it can help alleviate anxiety and nervous exhaustion, it deepens the breath. It is also useful for excessive perspiration.

Rose (Rosa damascene)

My clients have found this truly luxurious aroma helpful in restoring libido and re- building self-confidence. It can be used to help improve the condition of mature sensitive skins.

Clary- sage (salvia sclarea)

A deeply relaxing and stress- relieving oil that can help to ease anxiety and nervous tension whilst uplifting the spirit. It blends well with lavender, geranium, bergamot and other citrus oils.

Aromatic waters are also effective in helping menopausal conditions. They are uplifting, cooling, refreshing and can be carried in a spritzer spray to combat hot flushes or power surges during the day.

Bitter orange flower water has a sedative action and is traditionally used for anxiety. It can also be used as a skin tonic- it has moisturising and rejuvenating properties it can help to improve the dry skin that many menopausal women experience.

Below is a brief summary of two treatments I conducted for menopausal clients whilst working with a group of Doctors at their practice in Chorley.

Woman aged 54 years.

Symptoms - tension headaches, stress, difficulty sleeping, arthritic knee, constipation and varicose veins.

Current medication- HRT patches. (Doctors permission received) Selected oils - lime blossom macerated oil (antispasmodic effect/ sedative effect), vetiver, Ylang Ylang, benzoin and clary-sage. The oils were blended with white base lotion to be applied nightly to the upper body and during the day to the abdomen and legs.

Result - better sleep, fewer tension headaches, stress and anxiety reduced. Circulation improved due to application of lotion to the legs. Over all the client felt refreshed and more balanced.

Woman aged 60 years.

Symptoms - hot flushes, night sweats also occurring during the morning, anxiety and depression.

Current medication- none, GP referred her immediately for aromatherapy treatment.

Selected oils - bergamot, geranium and rose. These were blended in a white base lotion to be applied to the upper body after a morning shower. A second blend of Frankincense, sandalwood and Ylang Ylang with base oil was provided for the client to apply before bed.

Result-the day time anxiety and night sweats quickly diminished but she still experienced the night sweats. I therefore changed the evening blend to Petitgrain, Neroli and rose, blended in white base lotion and sweet almond oil. This brought a reduction to the frequency of night sweats.

The medical profession are beginning to realise how effective aromatherapy can be especially where modern medicine has been unable to help. By empowering ourselves with the pleasant use of aromatherapy blends and natural ingredients we can bring greater balance and significantly improve our health and wellbeing.

Chapter 7

Aromatherapy in the Home

Home is where the heart is. It should be our own personal sanctuary, a place of comfort and bliss. Our own little part of the world where we can truly be ourselves.

Every home has its own smell or aroma. It's hard to recognise this ourselves because we become accustomed to it but others will notice it. We can ensure that our home has a pleasing aroma by using essential oils. My good friend Kay has a home scented with lemongrass and citronella. Whenever I smell these aromas it reminds me of Kay's last home which was a welcome hub for the many friends who frequented her kitchen for a chat and to share tea and sympathy. Kay is a healing guru and her home was a reflection of her. You felt well just being there. Your home can be in harmony with you by using similar aromas to your favourite fragrances and scented candles. Aromatherapy is healing to the body mind and spirit and it is so simple to create a healing home with aroma. Let us start at the entrance.

As people walk through the door they can bring energy/vibes into your home. They may have wiped their feet on your door mat but they still bring the baggage from their day with them in the form of energy. To ensure that any negativity is left behind and to cleanse them of excessive emotional baggage, sprinkle Juniper berry essential oil on your doormat Juniper has been known for protection since biblical times when it was said the Mary, Joseph and the baby Jesus hid behind a Juniper tree to escape from King Herrod who threatened their lives. It is also wise to do as Eastern cultures do and remove shoes before entering the home as your home is a sacred space and should be respected.

Once your guests enter they should be met with a fresh inviting fragrance. Something citrus for the day time is pleasing and uplifting. It lightens the mood and clears the head. Dropping a couple of drops of a citrus oil onto a smelling strip and placing it on a covered radiator or protected source of heat allows the molecules to evaporate slowly and fragrance the environment. In your living room you can do the same with your cushions, unzip the cover and slide the smelling strip inside. I use paper leg waxing strips which I cut into strips to use as smelling strips. If you have curtains, then slide smelling strips into the hem, every time you open the curtains you will be greeted with fragrance. Re apply drops of oil every 3 days to the strip.

The kitchen is a great place for using essential oils. Mopping your floor can be an aromatic experience with the cooling anti- bacterial properties of eucalyptus globulus.

Adding essential oil that is close to its use by date to a bucket of hot water is a great way to cleanse the floor of your home and use up essential oils that you may have had for a long time. On a clean dish cloth add a few drops of tea tree or lemon and wipe your work surfaces and sinks. This will give a fresh antiviral atmosphere.

If you have a study or work room, refreshing peppermint oil will keep you mentally alert and keen to study. Use 4 drops in a burner (follow the instructions on the leaflet that comes with the burner). Never allow the burner to run dry. If you don't have burners use a bowl of warm water and add the scented peppermint oil. Rosemary is equally effective for concentration but don't use if you have high blood pressure or epilepsy as these conditions are contra-indicated to its use.

The dining room is the place to eat and share conversation with friends and family. In Victorian times the ceiling rose was above the dining table and signified that whatever was discussed at the table was held in confidence. Ceiling roses are still popular in many homes. Rose therefore would be a pleasing loving aroma for family get together. Heartfelt conversations and loving family meals. Bergamot essential oil is also useful for stimulating the appetite and controlling it. Bergamot is in earl grey tea so you may already be familiar with its aroma. Vaporise these oils in the room. Or use natural based scented candles at the dining table. Warming digestive stimulating ginger, clove and cinnamon can also be vaporised in the dining room, reminding us of warm apple pie and Christmas.

The sitting room is a relaxing gathering place for most families so this room can be fragranced with Frankincense and Petitgrain. These aromas relax the body and mind and remove anxiety. Geranium is also another harmonising aroma for a family home. Lavender and Geranium create a soothing, balancing atmosphere, whilst uplifting the emotions and reducing stress.

The bedroom is a place we go to for sleep and to enjoy intimate loving experiences. To aid sleep Lavender, Clary sage and Sandalwood will still the mind and gently lull us into a deep replenishing sleep. Always avoid alcohol when using Clary sage as a combination of the two can bring on night mares. To create a more romantic atmosphere the heady exotic oils can be chosen such as Jasmine, Rose and Neroli or Ylang Ylang. These oils have aphrodisiac properties and are deeply arousing. Use the oils blended with floral waters to create pillow sprays or vaporise them a couple of hours before bed, but never leave an oil burner candle lit whilst you sleep. Always blow out the candle before you go to bed.

Cleanse your room in the morning with a refreshing room spritz of grapefruit and juniper to clear the air and deodorise the environment. Grapefruit is revitalising and Juniper berry is cleansing and clearing.

Aromatherapy can make your home a more relaxing and healing environment. It can help us to express our individuality and share our fragrance preferences with those we invite in.

Chapter 8

Aromatherapy and oral hygiene

Coming from a background in beauty therapy, I became interested in Aromatherapy during my teacher training in the late 1980's. I expected Aromatherapy to enhance my work but not to the extent to which it has. The benefits of this wonderful therapy to clients, friends and family have been astonishing. Aromatherapy has opened many new doors and touched my life in so many ways. Aromatherapy is for anyone and everyone, and so when I was asked by the British Dental Association to present a lecture on the benefits of Aromatherapy in Dental care I thought why not. I believe that Aromatherapy is beneficial in all areas of well-being and so I went along and delivered my lecture. The use of aromatic substances goes back thousands of years. Early civilisations recognised the therapeutic value of natural plant material. They captured the properties in unguents and lotions which were used to preserve everything from wood to bodies - as in mummification. Aromatics were part of everyday life - luxury, vanity, ceremonial and medicinal. Even today just think about how important fragrance/ perfume/ aroma is in our everyday life.

With Aromatherapy, aroma takes on a whole new meaning. Aromatherapy is the controlled use of essential oils which are natural extracts from aromatic plants obtained by distillation. The aim of Aromatherapy is to balance and harmonise the body and mind, it is a complementary therapy and not an alternative. This is where its strength lies, in its ability to work with orthodox medicine and the individual being treated. Aromatherapy has a supportive role and being a simple therapy it can be used by the patient/client as part of the care plan.

Essential oils can play a supportive role in dental health and hygiene - but it must be emphasised that with Aromatherapy essential oils are not taken internally (ingested) other than may be used in a mouth wash. Essential oils must be respected, as we do with other dental preparations and medicines.

One of the most beneficial essential oils for oral care is Myrrh; reference is made to this ancient oil in the bible. Myrrh is marvellous for keeping the gums healthy. It has healing properties where ulcers are present and is best used in a mouth wash for problem gums.

Recipe.

2 drops of Myrrh
20 mls of alcohol vodka

Add two drops of the above to a tumbler of fresh water and rinse the mouth. 2x daily. Tea tree which I am sure you are familiar with is another excellent essential oil for oral hygiene. It is a natural antiseptic and anti-viral agent. It can be used as above for a mouth rinse and as a gargle for a sore throat. Always obtain your essential oils from a reputable supplier as only high grade organic or wild crafted essential oils will provide the best results.

Other essential oils for dental care include Rose Otto; this beautiful oil can be used in a mouth wash for ulcers and gingivitis. It has anti- inflammatory properties.

Chamomile Roman is pain relieving and can be diluted in base oil such as Grape seed and applied externally to the cheek or jaw for toothache. A visit to the dentist can be a stressful experience for many people so Lavender inhaled from a tissue can be most useful for calming anxiety. The citrus oils such as Grapefruit can also reduce anxiety and provide a welcome fragrance, hiding the anti-septic clinical smell of the dental surgery.

Chapter 9

Cleopatra's beauty secrets

Cleopatra is renowned for her beauty, portrayed in more recent times by Elizabeth Taylor in Anthony and Cleopatra. But was she a real beauty? Historical silhouettes on ancient coins would have us believe that she was not as beautiful as we are told, but non the less this Egyptian Princess with Greek heritage has mystified man kind and conjured up fantasies of a goddess in human flesh, a seductress and exotic beauty like non before or after. She certainly had what it takes to seduce two very powerful men, Anthony and Caesar. What was it about her? Was it her knowledge and use of exotic oils and unguents, her beauty regime and her extravagance in perfuming her barges and palaces?

We are aware of the power of aroma and its effect on the olfactory bulb and how pleasant smells can stimulate the body and mind with a powerful narcotic effect. Was she then an aromatic enchantress, or an early Aromatherapist?

She rose to fame at 19 when she became Queen; with her Greek and Egyptian ethnicity she would have had exotic looks and olive skin. Lustrous hair would also have been part of her genetic inheritance so what a good start. Apparently only 30% of our good looks can be accounted for from the gene pool the rest is down to how we look after ourselves and our inner and outer beauty regime. So what were Cleopatra's beauty secrets?

As women we adore perfume, no women goes on a date without using her favourite fragrance. Perfume gives us confidence and there is nothing more alluring than a confident woman. Cleopatra knew this! She was a bathing beauty, her bath would have been laden with milk and honey both known for their favourable effect on the skin. Both are cleansing and exfoliating with mildly anti-septic properties. Rose and Frankincense would have fragranced the bath chambers. The Greeks, Romans and Egyptians were avid users of rose petals and Cleopatra loved rose petals. Young children walked before her in precessions scattering petals for her to walk on. Frankincense was highly prized by the Pharaohs of Egyptian times to. It was an expensive and highly prized commodity. Its smoke rising as a gift to the gods, only the kings and queens of Egypt could afford it. Its rich aroma would have filled the air.

To replicate Cleopatra's bath try the following;

1 cup of milk
1 cup of honey
5 drops of rose essential oil
3 drops of Frankincense essential oil.

We all know the value of regular exfoliation and Cleopatra certainly would have done. It's part of every girl's beauty regime. To keep her skin soft and youthful she used mineral rich salt from the sea and ancient river beds. It would have been almost pink in colour. She could have used the deep dark fertile mud from the banks of the river Nile as a body and face mask. Its dark organic properties, cleansing, purifying and balancing. The ancient olive, still highly prized today would have given forth its emerald oil to protect and nourish her skin, blended with the fragrance of incense. The temples and palaces oozed aroma as cosmetics were made for the queen of Egypt. Cedarwood was a popular tree of the day; its oil is circulatory and strengthening to the skin. It was used copiously by the Egyptians. The wood of barges were said to be made and preserved with cedar and the sales soaked in rose water. The Nile would have been fragrant in those days.

Cedar wood resin was used to embalm the dead and extracts of cedar would have been used in perfumes and preparations for the living.

To exfoliate like Cleopatra, try this recipe.

1 cup of sea salt
Half a cup of olive oil
5 drops of Cedarwood oil.

Historical pictures of ancient artefacts recovered from temples and pyramids show pedicure tools and pumice stone. Open sandals and marble floors would have encouraged the need for regular foot care and painting the nails with henna for adornment was common practice. The heels of the feet may have been extremely dry and cracked due to the heat.

Thick unguents and cream like base solutions would have been prepared to combat the dry cracking skin. These potions combined with aromatic extracts of benzoin, spikenard and even lavender, which was popular in Roman times would have been massaged into the feet for both pleasure and remedial purposes. To prepare an aromatic foot treatment for yourself, try the following recipe.

Cracked feet cream

60 gram of base cream
10ml wheat germ oil
5 drops of Benzoin
5 drops of Lavender
5 drops of Spikenard.

Being women of great reputation and responsibility Cleopatra knew how to care for her body. It is said that "her hair was redolent of myrrh" and each part of her body anointed with a different perfume!

To create a Hair tonic blend try the following;

2 drops of Sweet Thyme essential oil
2 drops of Himalayan Cedarwood
3 drops of Rosemary

3 drops of Lavender
30 ml Jojoba oil
20 ml Grape seed oil.

Massage a small amount into the hair each night, leave for at least 1 hour. Try this for 2 weeks.

For facial care Cleopatra would have used milk and honey to cleanse and masks of milk, honey, yeast and clay would also have been used. For puffy eyes, masks made of ripe avocado would have been applied. The Persian face mask was also popular. You can prepare this yourself with egg yolk and olive oil. Apply to the skin for 20 minutes and then rinse off. Tone with rose water and moisturise with a blend of Sweet Almond oil, rose and Frankincense.

For breast care vetiver, sweet fennel and geranium in a base of sweet almond oil would have supported the breasts and kept them firm and shapely. For body massage, which would have been offered daily, a similar blend of sweet almond and olive oil with orange and sweet basil extract would ease both body and mind.

We need to build regular massage into our lives and begin to appreciate how special we are by following the example of the Queen of Egypt.

One thing that we can really learn from Cleopatra is how to preserve a sense of the sacred Feminine and use this to reclaim balance and harmony in our lives. Simple natural beauty regimes can re-establish the art of ritual which many of us have lost in our busy schedules and day to day work schedules.

Re- connecting with some ancient practices and some simple self-pampering can increase the feel good factor in our lives and sends a powerful self-affirmation that we are all Kings and Queens of our own destiny.

Chapter 10

The oils of love

All things are in harmony with each other wise lore teaches us this. Plants and herbs and all growing things correspond with the moon and the planets. We are one. Plants associated with the planet Venus (planet of love and beauty) are said to be the ones used in ancient love lotions and potions.

Plants provide a positive energy and give aid to natural forces allowing a favourable loving outcome.

Perfumes and fragrances delight our senses and allow us to stop for a moment and search through our memory tracking the fragrance through time to a familiar place, sensation or person in our past.

Our choice of fragrance can be a way of expressing our mood or our personality. It can also be a way of celebrating an occasion. There are fragrances we fell in love to. Fragrances that move us to tears, which produce laughter, joy and sadness. Perfumes are openers to deep memories.

Essential oils are chemical messengers that are powerful beyond belief. They are truly oils of love created by sunshine and Mother Nature. Without aroma where would we be a life without the fragrance the colour and the wonderful energy that plants, fruits and herbs bring.

Rose – is a passionate, sensual and gently erotic fragrance. Said to be the closest scent to the natural scent of a woman. Luxurious, warm and mysterious it enlivens the heart and allows the heart to give and receive love. It eases grief and restores faith and hope. It can help to heal emotional wounds from loss and rejection.

Jasmine – It is said the cupid's arrow was tipped with Jasmine. It can reawaken passion both physically and emotionally. Jasmine restores sexual confidence and allows us to reach our true potential. I have heard it said that If Rose is the Queen of oils then Jasmine is the King.

Neroli – This oil relaxes the nerves, it is uplifting yet calming. It stabilises the heart and mind. It aids sleep and restlessness. It is sensual and spiritual. It has the ability to restore hope and joy. It is intensely female. It is an aroma abundant with possibility.

Ylang – ylang is a component of many modern perfumes a unisex fragrance merging the masculine and feminine. It is said to release blocked sexual energy and reconnect us to our emotional, sensual nature. This could be why its blossoms are spread on the marriage bed of Indonesian couples. Ylang-ylang is a calming oil which can ease feelings of anxiety.

Bergamot – uplifting, happy and carefree is the message of this essential oil. Allowing us to let go of negativity and to feel more optimistic. A wonderful mood balancer.

Essential oils are truly love in a bottle when used in Aromatherapy they can help us to nurture ourselves and those we care for.

Always use following the advice of a professional Aromatherapist.

Chapter 11

Sense-ology - Treatments that touch deeper

If you are a Therapist do your treatments really stimulate your client's senses? Do you reach out and touch your clients on all levels of the Holistic spectrum? Do you feed their soul and create that empty yet sacred space where self healing can take place? I am sure you do, but let me take the time to remind you how you can provide a totally sensational experience for your clients that will leave them feeling totally replenished.

Getting to know your client is very important if you are going to provide an effective treatment, just like teachers need to know the learning styles of the learner in order to support and encourage the comprehension and retention of knowledge, we Therapists need to ensure that every aspect of the treatment is pleasing and acceptable.

Visual, auditory, kinaesthetic. What they see, what they hear, how they are touched, what they smell and what they taste and of course the 6th sense, finding that rapport, an empathetic compatibility and understanding of what they may be feeling on an inner level, being sensitive to their needs.

Let us begin.

Sight - the treatment room should be pleasing to the eye, the colour, the comfort and the luxury of the experience a sanctuary of calm professionalism. You should be dressed accordingly, well groomed and smiling giving your client your full attention. First impressions are lasting impressions. Certain client types will enjoy scenes of nature, candles, flowers these all add a pleasing appearance to the eye. A room free from clutter is also important I once read that "emptiness is infinitely satisfying to the human mind" so to some clients a minimalistic setting is best.

Smell - knowing your clients aroma preference and vaporising her favourite fragrance subtly in the room. For milder aromas floral waters vaporised in the room provide a hint of aroma. One thing that I have discovered is that morning people enjoy rose scented fragrances and night owls prefer more heady exotic aromas like Jasmine. Smell is individual get to know your clients preference and change fragrances depending on their moods and emotions as you review their record card regularly.

Taste - The client's skin will drink in the oil during a massage treatment. Ensure that your carrier/ massage oil is rich enough or light enough to satisfy the thirst of the skin type. Quench a dry skin with jojoba and rosehip oil to lock in moisture and support and restore collagen and elastin. Calendula and avocado oil can enrich your carrier oil and provide a soothing, calming base for more easily irritated skin types. At the end of a treatment offer iced water with lemon or ice cubes of rose water (used for heat exhaustion in India and an ingredient in Turkish delight). Herbal teas are thirst quenching and therapeutic and compliment the holistic ethos.

Sound- Music and Sound are very personal and very therapeutic. Having the right music to enhance relaxation is important. Your client may already have a personal preference, this you can explore during consultation. Using a bell or Chinese symbol gently, can quietly signify the start and end of the treatment and guide the client back to consciousness from a deeply relaxed state. A water feature in the room can add that special element of nature or a wind chime hung near to a window, a soft tinkle in the breeze.

Touch – It is truly a gift to be able to massage another and it is a gift we all have. Learning our skill and continually updating and developing ourselves professionally will allow us to become true masters of our craft. In the Ayurvedic system it is said that the Pitta client will enjoy a skilled massage by a highly trained therapist, they will enjoy being given self help tips and techniques that they can use themselves at home. The Vata client needs a warm cosy nurturing treatment. They need to be cocooned in the safety of the treatment room and although they often ask for a deep treatment this is not always what serves them best. Once more it is about knowing your client.

The Kapha client will experience sluggish circulation and lethargy. A stimulating and invigorating treatment will be best for their general well-being. Listening to the client and observing how they receive the treatment is the way to developing a sensitive touch. Allowing the client to relax and not engaging them in conversation during the process encourages a calm tranquil environment.

Rapport – Meeting the client on their level, gaining a professional affinity or kinship with the client is what really makes a treatment work. Rapport is a relationship of mutual trust and understanding and an agreement between two people. It is what brings about the synergy of all the above and makes your treatment truly special. It's finding that compatibility whilst maintaining the Therapist Client relationship. A good rapport is the beginning of a good treatment.

Chapter 12

Destination Provence

Well summer is here and it is time for me to have a short vacation from teaching. This year I wanted to do something special so when my friend Jonathan Hinde from Oshadhi UK rang to tell me about a wonderful opportunity to visit Provence on a study trip, I said yes immediately! There was no hesitation. Provence is one of my favourite places on this beautiful planet and July is Lavender season. In the past I have enjoyed many aromatic adventures in the high Alps of Provence and travelled the area in pursuit of excellent essential oils, knowledge and culinary delights. But the one place I have longed to visit was Malte Hozzel's place in Orto de Prouvenco close to Aurel. This is the venue for my studies. The title of the conference is "Plants and Man". Aromatherapy is one of those subjects that you just continue to learn, it is a "journey rather than a destination" as the saying goes and I am passionate about learning. I shall enjoy the food of Provence, I will spend time in prayerful meditation and I will learn more about essential oils and their therapeutic capabilities.

Orto du Prouvenco - means "large garden of Provence" the pays de Salt is one of the densest areas of medicinal plants in Europe. Such a fragrant environment filled with the fragrance of wild thyme and other herbaceous aromas. The regional cuisine is influenced by the abundant herbs of Provence plus ingredients such as Goats cheese, olives and garlic with a strong Mediterranean influence. These are among my favourite things. Provence is also the largest wine region specialising in dry Rose wine.

I'm flying to Marseille via Paris and from here my adventure will begin.

Marseille is the second largest city in France and one of the oldest. It was first discovered by the Greeks and used as a trading port. It is the capital of Provence.

I travel onwards to Aurel and "Orto" this is where we will begin with a botanical walk to collect medicinal plants for distillation. During the week I will be visiting the Gorges de la Nesque, Mount Ventoux on a botanical excursion and an organic distillery.

There is also a Lavender Museum at the Abbey of Senanque. The abbey is a 12th century working Abbey. In front of the Abbey is a valley of Lavender fields which will be in full flower and ready for harvest in late July-August. I am looking forward to capturing this on camera and breathing in its fragrant beauty.

A visit to the Salagon Priory is also scheduled to take in the ethno-botanical gardens. The Conservatoire is said to be an ethnological museum and presents some beautiful flowers and aromatic plants of the region.

The name Provence came from the fact that the region was the first Roman province outside of Italian territory therefore the Romans called it "our province" and so the area became 'Provence' to the French.

Provence has mostly a Mediterranean climate, dry summers and mild winters. The Mediterranean sun in the south of France is the reason we have so many aromatic plants exist in the area. The essential oil is the plants protection against high levels of heat. Hence we have fragrance and perfume! Grasse (a town high in the south of France as you may know?) was known as the perfume capital of the world. Where fragrant blossoms were grown for the perfume Industry. Grasse is a great place to visit with its perfume houses and fragrance museums.

Apparently because the Ice-age glaciers didn't reach the Mediterranean; many plants did not spread to the North when the glaciers melted. This left many species of plants in specific locations. The area where I am studying is abundant with medicinal plants!

The trees of Provence are very distinctive with a wide variety of Pine and Oak, but the most typical of all in the area is the Olive tree! Apparently olives have been grown in Provence for over 2500 years. There is so much history to the olive tree dating back over 6000 years and fossils discovered in Santorini provide evidence of the olive trees existence over 60,000 years ago. Its origins are thought to be in the Middle East. Historically it has been described for use in many religious traditions. Jewish, Christian and Muslim faiths favoured the olive. One of the many interesting things we know about olive oil is its benefits in skin care, but have you ever used it as a cleanser? The Romans certainly did before soap was invented. Olive oil has so many health benefits and as an Aromatherapist I have started to use this oil more in my practice and in the preparations I make for skin care. The Mediterranean diet rich in olive oil and tomatoes has been clinically proven to help prevent skin damage from sun exposure. I myself took part in this research some years ago. The findings confirmed that a diet rich in tomatoes and olive oil certainly delay the ageing process.

Aurel is the village where I am staying. It is a beautiful village with steep streets which appear to be carved out of the rock. In the background is the white peaked Mount Ventoux and surrounding the Village are valleys of Lavender. The main growing area for lavender fields in Provence are around the foot of Mount Ventoux and the Gordes. It blooms from the last week in June until the beginning of August when harvest time begins. So July is the best time to absorb the Lavender fields in all their glory. I am sure that you know the benefits of

INSPIRATIONAL AROMATHERAPY

Lavender essential oil as it is such universal oil with so many therapeutic properties and the French Lavender in my opinion has a superior quality due to the altitude it is grown at.

The majestic Sun flowers are also in full bloom, their faces to the sun. The contrast of Lavender and golden yellow is amazing. I remember the picture from my last visit to Provence.

The flight to Marseille was smooth. It was a delight to meet my greeter Axil and the delegates from Prague who gave me a warm welcome. It was a long car ride from the airport to Sault and then onto Aurel but as we left the auto route the vine fields and lavender was a welcome sight. The sunflowers had bowed their heads in the fading sun light. As we wound around the mountain roads we saw the breath-taking patch work of mauve and shades of green as the beautiful lavender fields blended with the provincial farm land. The view of Aurel nestling in the mountain side was a delightful sight and as we left the road onto a mountain track barely passable by car we landed in a heavenly location surrounded by lavender and butterflies. High in the Alps away from the bustle of life our aromatic adventure begins.

My room is surrounded by open field and insects. The cicadas (cigals) are musical. The path to the main house along a mountain track gives excellent views of sheer natural beauty like I have only ever found in Provence.

Breakfast outside the main house is international only one other from the UK. It's already very hot at 8am. I am surrounded by lavender and butterflies its magical.

Our lecture begins with Malte giving us a tour of the aromatic plants around the house. Blue cypress - strong and powerful ketone rich oil which should be used carefully as with all oils high in ketones, but highly mucolytic, I had come across the blue cypress on my visits to Australia many years ago. It was being re- introduced there in 1998. The Blue Cypress here is a different variety.

Yarrow - this plant was everywhere. It produces a blue oil rich in chamazulene giving it anti-inflammatory properties.

Lavender - or more precisely Lavandin, It is grown for its ease in farming and its high quality yield. It was cultivated as a cross between true Lavender and spike Lavender. This is grown a lot in the area as it is a hardy plant. There are also many varieties of mint in Provence, the mountain mint is a small hardy plant with tiny pink flowers it is ketonic. The field mint which is a lager plant grows profusely. Peppermint oil is the coldest oil we are told, it triggers our skin receptors into the sensation of cooling. It is also a very powerful pain killer.

Melissa - lemon balm is another of the lamiaceae family growing abundantly around the region. It has a lemon scented aroma yet it looks like mint. A Beautiful and expensive oil due to the labour intensive extraction. Melissa means "honey bee" and it certainly attracts the bees. An interesting fact that Malte our teacher told us was that the temperature of the beehive is the same as human blood!

It's amazing the power of nature and as we continued to explore the aromatic plants at Orto we began to discuss Neroli (orange blossom).

Neroli contains neral an aldehyde. Neroli is very powerful healing oil. It aids Sleep and is soothing to the nervous system. It is also indicated for aiding in the healing of Crones disease?

Finally before lunch we discover and discuss the Norway spruce. This tree produces an excellent energy restoring essential oil. Indicated for fatigue or when you have flu. The conifers are the lungs of the planet and aid respiratory conditions.

The sun is very hot even in the early morning so after 3 hours of lecture it is time for a welcome lunch.

After lunch we collect wild lavender using the traditional scythe to cut it low down so that the plant will grow well the following year. We carry it to the still and distil the oil from the lavender. Within a couple of hours we have the precious essential oil and the divine hydrolat. I was surprised how little time it took to produce. I have seen lavender distillation on many occasions and helped to load the still but to actually collect and extract was quiet an experience.

Later in the day we drove to Brante to get some excellent views of the majestic Mount Ventoux. I cannot believe how beautiful this area is. The landscape is phenomenal. We drink coffee and share aromatic stories in Brante in a tiny cafe that looks like it has been built into the mountain side.

On our return to the car we hear the choir in the tiny chapel and the church bells ring.

Winding our way back towards Aurel we see the lavender fields once more and smell the aroma of Provence. It's a magical place the atmosphere is so restorative.

Arriving back at Orto I walk back to my chalet accompanied by Junko (from Japan) and Stephanie (from Berlin) along the mountain path we see the shadows of the mountains and as it gets dark we need the torch light. France has reintroduced the wolf back into the area and there is always the possibility of wild boar so we tread with caution. The chalet is only 10 minute walk away. The night sky is amazing and although the area is very remote we feel safe. Wild boars don't usually appear until September and although we hear the wolves we don't see them!

There is a great thunderstorm in the night with lightening and power cuts it is terrifying as the rain hammers down and it is like a scene from a horror film. But these wonderful extremes in weather condition are the reason for the abundance of plants from the Lamiaceae family.

Monday morning is shrouded in mist creating a beautiful scene and a fresh coolness in the air. Many of our companions have taken the opportunity to partake in Chi-gong. Chi -gong is based on a series of movements to enhance well-being and bring peace and calmness to the body and mind. The lesson begins at 6 am at the back of the house in the open fields.

Our morning lesson is the spirituality of plants and some interesting presentations of rare plant oils and production in India.

A fascinating morning so informative.

After a fabulous lunch of fresh Mediterranean cuisine salads and fish and goat's cheese and beautifully cooked tofu, fresh fruits and herb teas, we set off to climb Mount Ventoux. We steadily drive the shear mountain roads with views that appeared to be out if a fairy tale. Patch work natural pictures of shades of mauve and green. Vine yards and cherry orchards interspersed with Lavender and Lavandin. We stopped on route to admire wild fennel growing at the road side and photograph the scenery. As we wound our way up the mountain we came across cedar wood, pine and fir trees creating a majestic cathedral of nature. The young pine trees have long double stemmed needles, the cedar has its needles in star like bunches and the fir trees have smooth thick needles that look and feel soft and fur like. This enabled us to identify many of the beautiful trees. Close to the summit at about 1,000 metres we found spike lavender and smelt it's camphorous leaves. Helichrysum was clinging to the rock face with its spices curry like aroma and Cade a variety of juniper with its purple berries covered the road side. We saw wild mountain thyme and alpine herbs such as harebell. In the back ground the sheep could be heard by their tickling bells around their necks. At the summit the view was like looking out from Heaven on Gods kingdom. Never before have I seen such scenery and nowhere in earth could such beauty exist! It was like a scene from the lord of the rings. The temperature at the summit was 11 degrees! As we descended it rose to 21 degrees.

We drive back to Aurel for dinner of white pumpkin grown in Provence in coconut oil, salad and a selection of local cheeses. Local Rose wine and excellent conversation. Another wonderful day of learning and sharing knowledge and enthusiasm for aromatic plants.

Tuesday we wake to the sun. This will be another hot day the freshness from the recent storm still retains a pleasant breeze but it is early and there is time for the sun to heat up the day. Ilyas one of the delegates from Tunisia finds Green myrtle growing on the land. Its name comes from the Goddess Myrtea of purity. Myrtus communis vert is good for respiratory conditions and is gentle enough for asthmatics. Massaged on the chest and upper back it eases congestion and aids breathing. I often purchase this oil when I visit Provence.

The morning we spend looking at the chemistry of essential oils and the different chemical families.

We inhale the oils and appreciate their molecular structure. We study the various therapeutic properties of the chemical compounds it is a fascinating morning. After lunch of salmon pasta and fresh Provencal salad we set off for Salagon which is a monument and museum gardens. Salagon is in Mane. We pass some fabulous lavender fields where we stop for photographs and to inhale the sweet perfume. We find a lavender field whose comfortable beds have been invaded by daisy like flowers which we initially mistake for chamomile but soon realise it is not. It makes a great photo opportunity however. When we arrive at the aromatic gardens we see an array of plants that we have merely read about but now in their natural glory but not in their natural habitat. We see patchouli, vetiver, verbena and calendula to name but a few. Malte talks about each one as we walk through the fragrant garden. We find pelargonium tomontosum which I have not come across for many years.

Wednesday we are up early. The sky is deep azure blue. Not a cloud in the sky. We have breakfast and set off for the Market in Sault.

We also are set to visit an organic Lavender distillery.

Sault is busy it is market day and there are an array of colourful stalls selling beautiful clothes and aromatic gifts. We have 2 hours to peruse the markets before we set off for the distillation plant.

Everyone returns loaded with bags and happy faces. Lavender honey and body lotion fragranced with mountain herbs. Junko my friend buys a beautiful basket almost as big as herself.

We set off for the organic distillery this is where Oshadhi get their lavender oil. The whole process is demonstrated to us and we watch helichrysum distilled. There is very little Helichrysum grown in France and its price is very high. As we leave the distillery we find another local grower who is distilling Lavender. They are not organic but use ecological methods. I buy lavender soap.

Lunch is a picnic at le combette. Then we continue our aromatic studies on the chemistry of essential oils.

Thursday is a full day excursion to Roussillon the red village and gorge and to Gorde and the abbey of Senanque. It is an extremely hot day I am melting and the local insects have feasted on my body. Roussillon is beautiful and the path along the red gorge reminds me of Australia. The heat is intense but we get some fascinating pictures. Later we sit in a cafe and enjoy people watching.

The abbey is a beautiful sight as we descend the mountain along a winding road. The lavender surrounding the abbey is a beautiful sight. The abbey produce their own essential oils which I purchase and a few other Lavender memoirs. Some of the group wander the grounds; I go with a small party of people to sit in the cool abbey in meditative silence.

INSPIRATIONAL AROMATHERAPY

To soon it's time to return, but the day has been long and hot. We have time to shower and change and then our generous hosts have prepared a feast for the weary travellers. I'm wearing my lavender dress and Varsher from Prague calls me the Lavender Lady!

A nice evening yet again, we have become a group of friends and my Northern accent causes great amusement as the many nationalities try to impersonate me. Japan, German and Algerian versions of the Mancunian accent was highly amusing to me!!!!!

On our return to the chalet we see a star lit night like I have never experienced before. So many stars!!! It's amazing! with only the light from a mobile phone we see our first snake across the path. The sound of wolves as they have been reintroduced into France.

I am glad to find my room and I'm happy the centipede in residence is settled near the door and not in my bed. A wonderful day of beauty and good company. Good food, wine and heavenly surroundings.

Friday is a full day of lecture. We have so much information to cover. Aromatherapy and carrier oils are the first topic. Although I have much knowledge it is always nice to get a different slant on the subject from another teacher. Malte has a very spiritual perspective which is interesting and some of which resonates with my own beliefs and feelings about the aromatherapy.

We revisit the work of many famous authors and their suggestions for blending from a chemical basis. Franchome and Penoel among the authors. I studied aromatology with Penoel in the 90's. I remind myself to dig out my notes upon my return.

We look at many different recipes and suggestions for blends. Later we continue looking for medicinal plants in the garden and find thyme linalol type, sage and juniper berry.

Saturday is our final day time is endless in Provence no beginning and no end just sheer natural rhythm of day and night. I have lost track of the days. We have the option of a late start and a day with Malte or we can visit Avignon? I choose to stay at la combette. We sit under the linden blossom and talk about the connection between plants and man and more importantly the essential oil connection. Integrated aromatic medicine is the way forward for the wise but will the world open its eyes to this concept? After lunch we take sencha tea with the small group who remained at home and we explore more of the land. Varsher one of the students from Prague has produced a wonderful presentation of our 9 days in Provence, as I watch it I feel moved by the beauty that she has captured and the memories we will share in the photographs she has taken. Later in the evening she will present the film to Malte, Fabien and the rest of la Combette house hold as a thank you for the exceptional hospitality they have shown us.

Before Dinner I, Stephania and Ilyas walk into Aurel and explore the small town. Aurel is the village close to where I am to be staying. It is a beautiful village with steep streets which appear to be carved out of the rock. In the background is the white peaked Mount Ventoux and surrounding the Village are valleys of Lavender. The main growing area for lavender fields in Provence are around the foot of Mount Ventoux and the Gordes. It blooms from the last week in June until the beginning of August when harvest time begins. So July is the best time to absorb the Lavender fields in all their glory. I am sure that you know the benefits of Lavender essential oil as it is such universal oil with so many therapeutic properties and the French Lavender in my opinion has a superior quality due to the altitude it is grown at.

We stop at a cafe and to my surprise meet a Father and Daughter who were originally from Blackburn two more northern folk in Provence?

We go back to la Combette for our final meal together for the next day we would start our journey home.

Back in the UK I reflect on the wonderful trip to Provence and how I long to share my experiences with my students and friends. I intend to return. I would love for you to join me.